»I truly enjoyed the flow and weave of words that spoke clearly about complex and fundamental aspects of life emerging on Earth in a body. I hear prosody of voice offering deeply lived experience, stated in ways that I can understand and receive from behind the words. I sense a silent understanding in my body as it changes in response as I read. The metaphor of tiny instruments appeals to me, describing a way of relating to our own patterned behaviour and its impact on relationships to others. The drawings are a gentle nourishment that support the ideas.«

Caryn McHose

Movement Educator, Certified Advanced Rolfer, and Somatic Experiencing Practitioner

Author of *How Life Moves, Explorations in Meaning and Body Awareness*, Collaborator (with Andrea Olsen) for *Body Stories: A Guide to Experiential Anatomy*

»I found reading A Small Book of Big Ideas to be like a calming pause in an oasis, a brief respite from today's frantic world.«

David Moore, PhD

Professor of Psychology, Pitzer College and Claremont Graduate University

Author of *The Developing Genome: An Introduction to Behavioral Epigenetics*

A Small Book of Big Ideas: Reflections on a Conversation with Destiny

Raveen Kulenthran

Illustrated by Asta Caplan

Tiny Instruments Press
www.tinyinstruments.org

ISBN:
978-3-9824273-0-0 – E Book
978-3-9824273-1-7 – Paperback
978-3-9824273-2-4 – Hardcover

Illustrations by Asta Caplan

Cover and book design by Nerina Wilter

Introduction

This book may be of interest to anyone who wishes to experience their life a little differently. The narrative stimulates self-reflection that sheds light on the actions we need to take in order to chart a new trajectory for our lives. Each of us has a unique story – a tale that includes our struggles.

The book begins by unravelling the threads of our story into two categories: the threads that we have inherited and the threads that have been woven through experience. The latter entwine with the directives of family and society, so the narrative deviates briefly to paint a picture of the complexities pervading society. It uses this picture as context to emphasise the importance of compassion and kindness, and the need to work for the welfare of society, as we chart life's new trajectory.

After stressing that the re-charting of our life trajectory goes hand in hand with the betterment of society, the writing takes on a more practical tone. It introduces the philosophical essence underpinning Yoga and then overlays that essence onto the unravelled threads of story. The text uses philosophical metaphors as it gathers momentum towards the main message: how we may cultivate a sensitivity to the consequences of our actions.

I believe that such a sensitivity can be extremely revealing and rewarding. It acquaints us with the forces that conceal the essence of our existence – our soul – and it enables us to harness those forces to transcend the self-limiting legacies of our old story. This relationship with the invisible forces swirling around us empowers us to break with the past and begin to re-chart our life's trajectory.

Of course, the message communicated in this book does not pretend to be absolute truth. It is relative truth – my truth. It expresses thoughts distilled from my life experiences over the past four decades. The main events behind those experiences, and the sentiments I felt as I navigated them, are detailed in the Afterword.

Although the narrative derives from my own felt experiences in one way or other, I constructed my sentences to be somewhat neutral: I want the readers to be able to relate to the narrative with their own lives as context. To achieve the desired unbiasedness, I draw on principles from various disciplines: theoretical physics, genetics, epigenetics, neuroscience, manual therapy and spirituality. The books from which I extracted those principles are listed in the Bibliography.

I strove to accurately interpret the knowledge in those books and I expressed my deductions in suggestive language. I also tried to make my reasoning smooth and easy to follow. Where I have succeeded, I owe that success to the clarity and brilliance of the authors.

Where I have failed, the faults are mine, and mine alone to bear.

If this book helps its readers to see their lives from a different point of view, if it inspires them to take the steps needed to change their lives in positive ways, or even if it merely incites its readers to explore some of the books in the bibliography, then I would have overwhelming reason to feel rewarded.

Raveen Kulenthran
Munich, January 2022

1
A Wrinkled Crinkle

It is said that we were once tiny parts of an inconceivably dense and highly ordered singularity whose origins are a mystery. This conjecture is based on a theory formulated through the concerted efforts of observational deduction, rigorous calculations and creative experimentation. Whether or not the theory holds true, the insights derived from the aforementioned efforts – all of which confirm and reinforce one another – suggest that roughly 14 billion years ago, a singularity exploded with an unimaginable intensity. Chaos then ensued with unrelenting ferocity, throwing what was previously the singularity into the expansion of space and the stream of time – our universe.

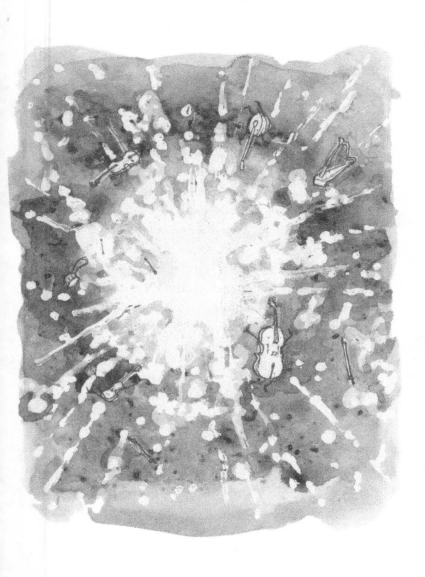

Fig. 1:
Singularity exploding with unimaginable intensity

Miniscule remnants of the earlier singularity, known as vibrations of matter and vibrations of force, are the basic ingredients of our universe. These vibrations – both near and far – interact among themselves through countless interactions arranged in a certain order. Although arranged in a particular order, each interaction is not uniquely responsible for any other. Rather, each interaction is interdependent with every other. The interactions also do not differentiate the past from the future, nor do they discriminate right from wrong. They just are. This suggests that the interacting vibrations may be presumed to be characterised by the quality of tranquillity.

Although characterised by the quality of tranquillity, at some point in time, interacting vibrations churned out additional qualities. How and why is unclear. What is clear is that the churning out of additional qualities transmuted vibrations into atoms that bonded with one another to become molecules, which, in turn, metamorphosed to arise as a myriad of emergent entities. These entities characterise our reality, a reality that is messy and complicated. This means that our universe can be comprehended on two layers – a fundamental layer, consisting of vibrations whose interactions are presumed tranquil, and an emergent layer, consisting of entities whose reality is messy and complicated.

The interrelationship between the two layers of our universe may be comprehended by visualising a crinkled fabric. The fabric as a whole represents the universe. The interweaving threads that comprise this fabric represent a substratum of interacting vibrations. And the crinkles that arise out of the fabric represent the emergence of entities. From the interconnectivity of the interweaving threads, we can appreciate that all vibrations in the universe are unified as one – the fundamental layer. From the arising of crinkles, we can appreciate that this unity can exude diversity through the emergence of entities – the emergent layer. Thus the crinkle in the crinkled fabric may be seen as a conglomeration of vibrations emerging from the unbroken wholeness of the universe.

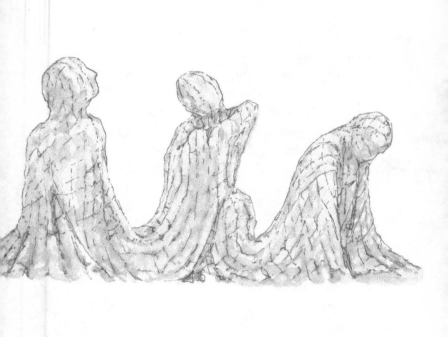

Fig. 2:
The two layers of our universe appreciated through the analogy of a crinkled fabric

Upon their emergence, crinkles interact differently from their encompassing vibrations. They interact through the laws of cause and effect. In obedience to these laws, when a crinkle carries out an act, whether conscious or seemingly insignificant, that act – through the interconnectivity of the fabric's threads – causes the fabric to form a wrinkle. This wrinkle affects many crinkles, prompting each crinkle into reactions that adopt aspects of the affecting wrinkle. In doing so, the crinkles become wrinkled crinkles. Thus wrinkled crinkles are a conglomeration of vibrations that, in emerging, shape and are shaped by actions and reactions that obey the laws of cause and effect. Among countless other things, wrinkled crinkles also include our bodies.

2

Inherited Story

Our story as a wrinkled crinkle arguably begins when a few remnants of the singularity that exploded collected together to form our planet, which was very hot at first. As planet Earth cooled, gases were emitted from its rocks, giving rise to an atmosphere. This early atmosphere enabled an environment that nurtured molecules to interact in such a way that basic lifeforms started to appear on Earth. These early lifeforms coordinated and aggregated themselves into cells and then – rather unhurriedly – evolved into numerous lineages of complex lifeforms. Among these many lineages, the lifeforms of one lineage – our evolutionary lineage – saw cells innovatively adapting their means of function so that entities in the form of humans emerged.

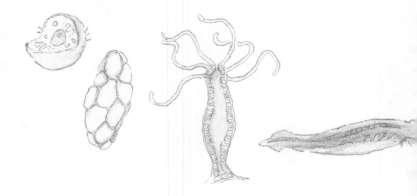

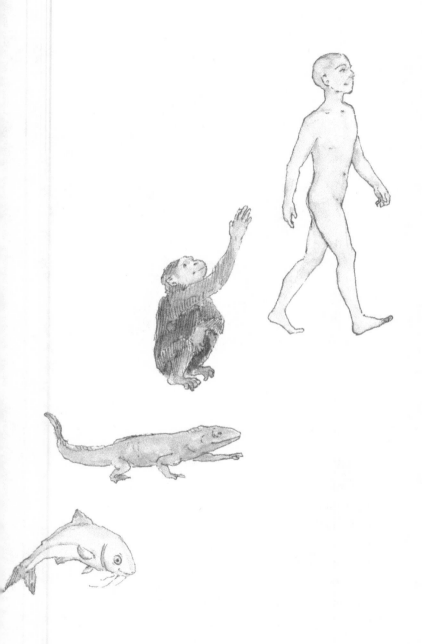

Fig. 3:
An abbreviated view of our evolutionary lineage

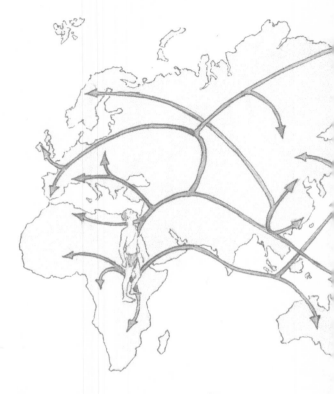

In finding themselves as human beings, our distant ancestors explored new frontiers, settling far and wide across our planet. Within and between their settlements, they formed families, embraced lovers, and at times, often through plunder and conquest, were perpetrators or victims of rape. By way of these events, humankind grew into an elaborate and entwining network of human bloodlines. Intriguingly, as those

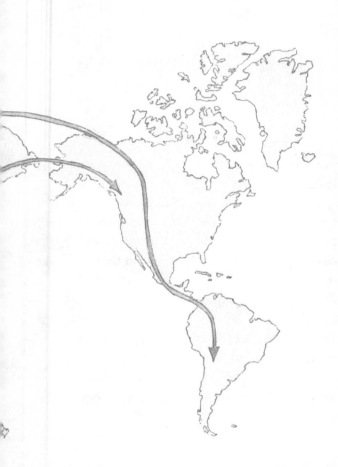

events – as well as events associated with our earlier evolutionary lineage – were unfolding, one remarkable molecule was surreptitiously conserving lessons associated with adaptations as an encrypted story. That molecule, found deep within our bodies, goes by the acronym "DNA". As we shall see shortly, it is also a purposeful molecule.

Fig. 4:
After emerging, our human ancestors explored new frontiers

The DNA molecule causes us to inherit the story of our evolutionary lineage and recent human bloodline by guiding our body's development. It does this through its own exquisite architecture, charming other molecules into decrypting that story and then courting those molecules into interactions that give rise to the cell – the smallest unit of life that can exist in our body. This invariably means that every cell in our body contains the same DNA molecule with the same inherited story. Period. Yet upon examination of our body, we encounter cells with diverse structures and functions. This suggests that there must be another factor contributing to the arising of the cell. There is. That factor is our environment.

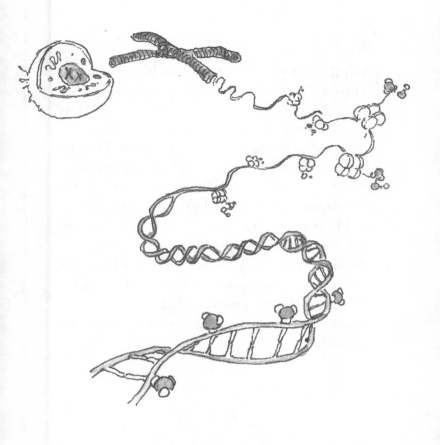

Fig. 5:
The DNA molecule facilitates the arising of our cells

Whether as a growing dot in our mother's womb or as a developing entity on planet Earth, our environment gets inside of us, permeating through our body's many hierarchies to infiltrate the architecture of our DNA. Upon infiltration, our environment regulates DNA's interaction with other molecules. Our environment influences *which* lessons within DNA's encrypted story are allowed to be decrypted by the other molecules as well as how DNA itself interacts with those molecules. This regulation by our environment enables the interaction between DNA and other molecules to give rise to the cells with diverse structures and functions that collectively make our body. Thus our body results from collaboration between our DNA and our environment.

Because our body is a collaboration between DNA and environment, we may suppose that the story we inherited through DNA, although a major part of who we are, does not predetermine our destiny. In other words, despite being born with a particular story embedded in our cells, we can, to a certain degree, influence the manifestation of that story as we live our lives. Accordingly, if – for whatever reason – we should feel unfulfilled with our life, perhaps desiring a somewhat different one, then, by virtue of our body being a collaboration between DNA and environment, we have the potential to re-chart our life trajectory by changing the circumstances of our environment. Alas, if only all this were as simple as it sounds!

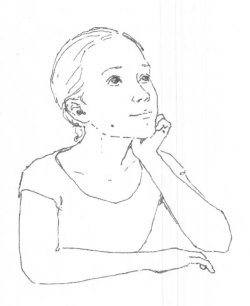

3
Experienced Stories

Each and every one of us has the potential to re-chart our life trajectory. This, however, is no stroll in the park. It is an arduous trek through a jungle. It is a trek that entails the likes of weeding out parasitic plants, the building of bridges over crocodile-infested swamps and the delving of channels between rivers, all the while politely keeping the leeches at bay and outsmarting the tigers attempting to sniff us out. Nevertheless, despite the arduousness of our trek, with intelligent preparation and a lot of heart, it can become a truly rewarding adventure. On this encouraging note, we prepare for the trek ahead by familiarising ourselves with the topography of the jungle we have to navigate through – our brain.

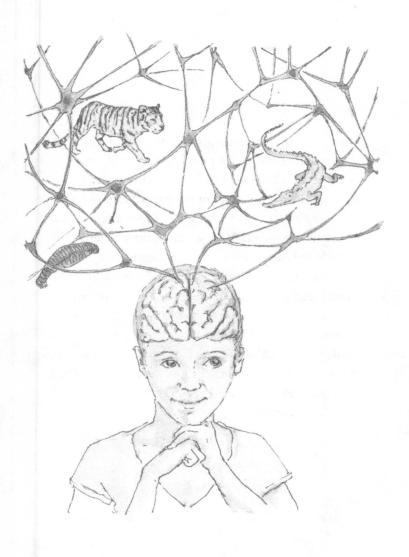

Fig. 6:
Navigating the workings of our brain can be likened to a trek through a jungle

Like the rest of our body, our brain – with its hills and valleys and elaborate neural rivers – arises through the collaboration between DNA and environment. Some of these rivers extend out of our brain and into our sense organs to capture the details of the circumstances of our environment. Among others, these details include the caring associated with our upbringing, the conditioning of our sociocultural training and the views of our intellectual schooling. These details are further sharpened or blurred by the books we've read, the movies we've watched, the music we've listened to, the conversations we've had, the jobs we've done, the people we've lived with, the countries we've visited, etc. The collective details captured by our senses to date are our experienced stories.

Our experienced stories influence how the rivers within our brain carve into its various hills and valleys and how these rivers associate with one another to form a network. This network moulds the finer aspects of our brain as we develop. This means that our brain's structure is a product not only of our inherited story, which manifests through the collaboration of DNA and environment, but also of our experienced stories, which are acquired through the details of the circumstances of our environment. And here lies a central point: our brain serves up a narrative that interweaves both these stories. This narrative – also known as "the voice in our head" – interprets our every sensation. Because interpretation of sensation is perception, the narrative of our brain causes us to perceive the world not as it is, but as per our stories.

The narrative of our brain also imbues our body's conduct, steering the way we comport ourselves through life. As the narrative has a fair share of its origins in our experienced stories, our conduct reflects those stories more often than not. This is consequential. It causes us to behave in such a way that we unwittingly gravitate towards future experiences that are not dissimilar to our experienced stories, putting us in a vicious cycle that frustratingly impedes our ability to change the circumstances of our environment – a change pivotal to re-charting our trajectory. Fortunately there is a way around this impediment. This way lies in the fact that the finer aspects of our brain are malleable, open to the prospect of being gently restructured.

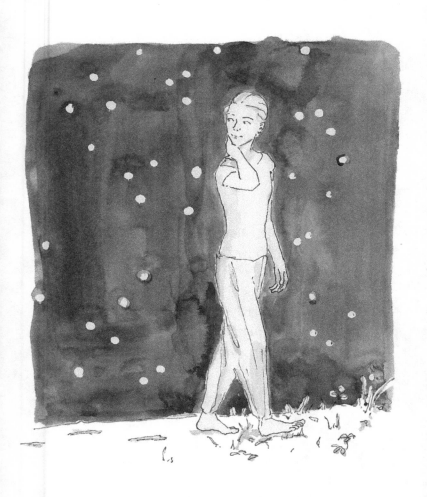

Fig. 7:
The narrative of our brain tends to steer us towards future experiences
that are not dissimilar to our past experiences

By virtue of our brain's malleability, we may coax its rivers into forming new associations and entice their flow to discover caverns of treasure deep within its hills and valleys. These efforts can result in a new narrative being served up – one that may perhaps create tectonic shifts in our conduct, steering us towards new and beautiful experiences that, in turn, may serve to re-chart our trajectory. Such efforts, however, require that we rise above the prevailing narrative by acting constructively, with persistence and self-reflection, and that we do so with an in-depth awareness of the circumstances of our environment. Let us digress briefly on this last point to inform ourselves about that which affects the circumstances of our environment – society.

4
Society

We live on a beautiful planet. It is a planet where majestic mountains tower over rainforests rich with innumerable lifeforms that, in turn, live off mighty rivers that drain into seas full of mysterious depths. It is also a self-sustaining planet, capable of ensuring we are comfortably fed and sufficiently clad as it replenishes itself. Sadly, however, as our network of humanity was growing and innovating, we took our planet's goodwill for granted, scrambling for its resources to pursue soulless materialism and unneeded consumption. Blinded and warped by our selfish and greedy desires, we became accustomed to measuring the quality of our lives by the quantity of our material wealth. The insatiability of such absurdity led us to revere senseless opulence. This, tragically, has caused our planet to be grotesquely raped.

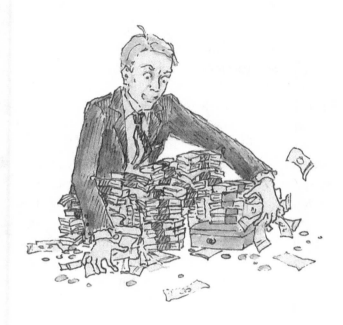

Fig. 8:
We are consumed by our selfish and greedy desires

The tragic violation of our planet has had catastrophic effects. Diverse rainforests became perverse plantations. Mighty rivers became silty floods. Clean air became poisonous gas. The list goes on. The consequences of such events mean that today we find ourselves in a world where complexities are not only adding up, but also multiplying at an alarming rate. These ever-mounting complexities – compounded by the exasperating prevalence of religious and cultural bigotry as well as our own disconnectedness through gadgetries that are themselves inundated with inaccuracies – are straining our interactions with one another. This, unfortunately, has resulted in our humanity being not one of a cohesive society, but one that is segmented.

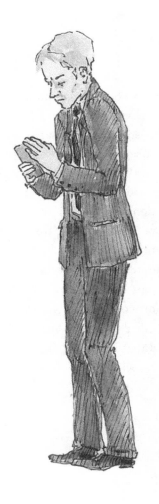

Fig. 9:
We are subjugated by our gadgets

Segmented, we have been unable to savour the beautiful fruits that could have grown from a harmoniously diverse society. Instead, we find ourselves drifting towards a particular identity, for example, a certain religion, culture or belief system. This might have been innocuous if we had not also forgotten our deeper, more common affiliations – to name just one, the fact that we all share a common ancestor. This forgetting of our common affiliations has meant that we have focussed on our petty differences. We became suspicious of the unfamiliar, which, over time, fermented an evil that brewed a form of political tyranny that has often resorted to abominable tactics, shepherding us into a bewildered herd that is fed lies. These falsehoods have infused fear into society.

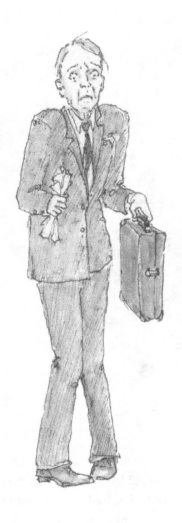

Fig. 10:
Greed has caused us to be in fear

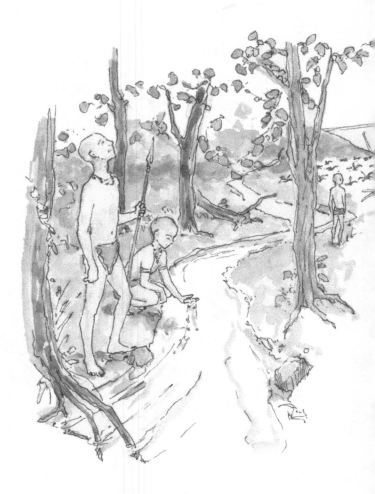

As fear is orchestrated by those who reign on a throne built and maintained by our greed, the most vulnerable of society are robbed of basic opportunities – food to eat, clothes to wear, water to wash with, light to read by, books to learn from, and meaningful work to do. This robbery has distressing consequences. Peaceful

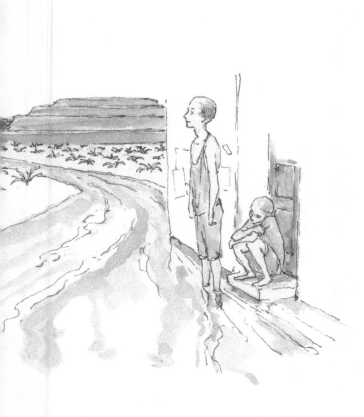

people become desperate criminals. Budding creativity becomes withering poverty. Preventable morbidity becomes premature mortality. The list goes on. Such tragedies tatter the social fabric of those affected, ruining any threads of hope they may have. Devoid of hope and deprived of opportunity to mend their tattered fabric, they are left with little choice but to resign their debilitated selves. Through no fault of their own, they silently suffer.

Fig. 11:
Greed and fear tatter the social fabric of the most vulnerable

Should we be fortunate and find ourselves in a part of the world where our eyes do not comprehend the tragedies of society, we may perhaps open our eyes to what is in front of us. To name just three: people who have been displaced, weather whose patterns have changed, and waste that hideously piles up. Such tragedies are also a consequence of greed and fear. Whether knowingly or unknowingly, our actions, through the far-reaching workings of cause and effect, have contributed to the calamities of our society. There is no escaping this hard truth. And, should we on the off chance, out of sheer vanity, be driving a fuel-guzzling monstrosity and doing so in a crowded city where public transport is a reliable amenity, then we are a bigger part of the problem than we may perhaps realise.

5

A Tiny Instrument

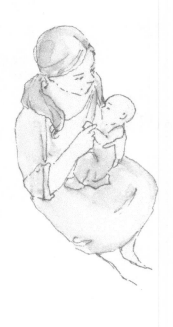

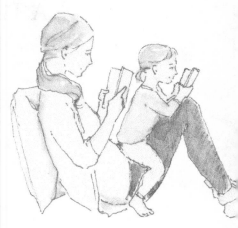

The preceding chapter saw us digressing to inform ourselves about the sombre state of our society. This was because society affects the circumstances of our environment, which – as was alluded to at the end of Chapter 3 – is the key to re-charting our trajectory. Furthermore, we are not sovereign entities. Rather, we are social entities obligated to one another – we needed to be given milk and touch to survive our earliest days on Earth. And as we grow, we imitate, interrelate and procreate, all of which are interactions. Thus, put succinctly, in being social entities that interact in an environment whose own circumstances are affected by the fabric of society, the re-charting of our trajectory demands that we are informed about society.

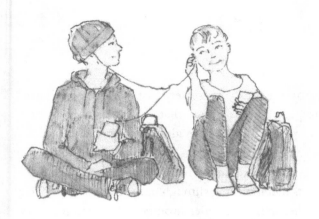

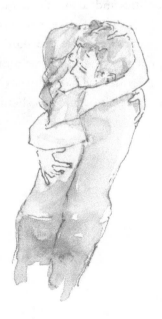

Fig. 12:
We are social entities obligated to one another

As social entities in a society that is not rosy, we have
a responsibility to ensure that our efforts to re-chart
our trajectory go hand in glove with the betterment of
society. Only through this responsibility do we have
a chance to contain the malignancy of greed and fear
that is metastasizing through our society, a malignancy
that lies at the root of environmental catastrophes,
abominable politics and economic inequality. This
responsibility, it is suggested here, may be shouldered
through the way we recognise one another and, in
particular, by encouraging harmony in the dynamics of
our interactions – because harmony has the potential
to resonate at a frequency that can shatter our greedy
desires and fearful aversions.

To encourage harmony into our interactions, we draw inspiration from the musicians of an ensemble. Deftly handling their respective instruments in relation to those of the others, the musicians collaborate by tuning in to one another, modulating the handling of their instruments to maintain the shared coordinative aim of playing a melody in harmony. Phrased succinctly, each musician sensitively harmonises with every other. While the dynamics of an ensemble can inspire our own ability to encourage harmony into our interactions, there is, however, one notable difference. Unlike these musicians, we do not handle an external instrument. We are the instrument. A *tiny* instrument.

As a tiny instrument, we harmonise by detecting
the subtleties of mannerisms and the peculiarities of
expression of those we interact with. Attention to these,
as well as to the pitch, timing and rhythm of any words,
equips us with the means to decipher the emotions in
their language, allowing us to tune in not to what they
are saying, but to what they mean. This, in turn, enables
us to evoke in ourselves a demeanour that may then
invite them to tune in to us. But despite our best efforts,
others may not always reciprocate. They may instead be
focussed on armouring and shielding themselves. As
unpleasant as this might be, in the spirit of harmony, we
should remind ourselves that there is far more suffering
than unpleasantness in the world. Their defence may
very well be due to suffering embedded in their unique
story.

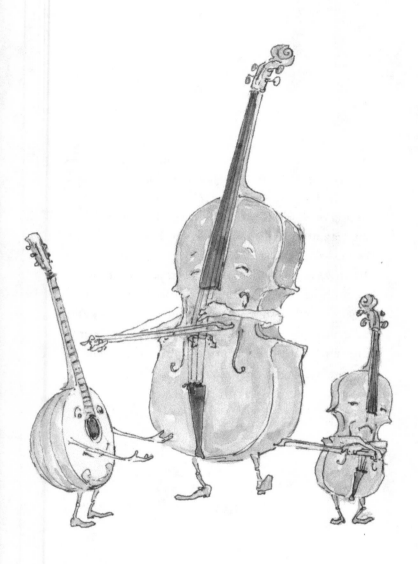

Fig. 13:
We harmonise by tuning in to the emotions of those we interact with

In viewing the other's defence as a hidden suffering, we may perhaps see reason to respond to their unpleasantness with compassionate kindness. This, nevertheless, requires strength – not the strength of flexing one's muscles, but the strength to weather unpleasantness. It is the self-composure necessary to be unshakable in stance, yet sensitive and adaptable to another's deep resonance. Such composure, however, can only be available to us if, prior to the moment when we call upon it, we have been meticulously and diligently mastering the tiny instrument that we are. The inhabitants of ancient India offer us a gradual but convincing way to cultivate ourselves.

6

A Leaf Out of India

India – a land that is home to a great ancient civilisation and one that has seen many cross migrations – is a country rich in numerous and diverse traditions. Among the many is Yoga. Although its exact origins are nearly impossible to pinpoint, it is said that its wisdom was consolidated by early inhabitants, who retreated into the peace and serenity of India's then-pristine forests. On entering the forest, in reverence of its natural splendour and out of gratitude for its shelter, they gave the forest respect. They did not erect boundaries around themselves, but instead grew with and into their surroundings, effectively harmonising with them. It was in this natural harmony that the wisdom of Yoga began to be consolidated.

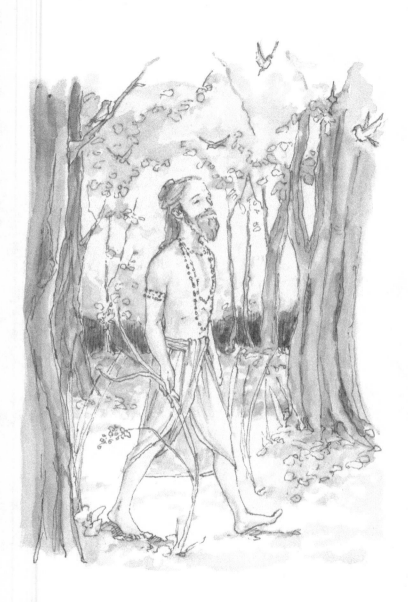

Fig. 14:
The wisdom of Yoga began to be consolidated in the peace and serenity of the forest

As the ancient inhabitants harmonised themselves with the forest, their sense of consciousness dilated, bestowing upon them the realisation that they were not separate from the forest. Through an unseen agency, they and the forest were one. Meditating on and contemplating this agency, and then contrasting their insights with the rich knowledge already prevalent in India at that time, these inhabitants – like modern-day champions of science – concluded that vibrations are the basic ingredient of the universe. Coming to vibrations in this way, they were able to describe our relationship with reality – which, the reader may recall from Chapter 1, is the emergent layer of our universe – with practical simplicity.

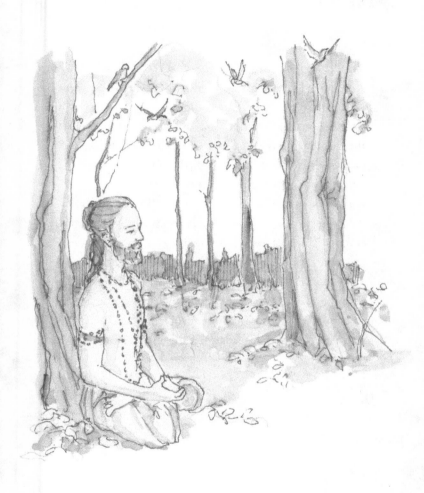

Fig. 15:
Consolidators of Yoga meditated and contemplated the universe in the forest

According to these early inhabitants, every miniscule
vibration in the universe is veiled in varying proportions
by three qualities: *tamas*, *rajas* and *sattva*. *Tamas* is
the quality of darkness, *rajas* is the quality of fire, and
sattva is the quality of light. If the quality of *tamas*
predominates in the veils of a conglomeration of
vibrations, the effect is sleepy lethargy. Conversely, if
the quality of *rajas* is in abundance, the effect is restless
activity. This suggests that when *tamas* predominates,
creation is doused, and when *rajas* is in abundance,
destruction is aroused. As one-sided as this may be,
through just a little of the third quality – the light of
sattva – *tamas* and *rajas* may be balanced in such a
way that the interplay between the three develops that
sattva.

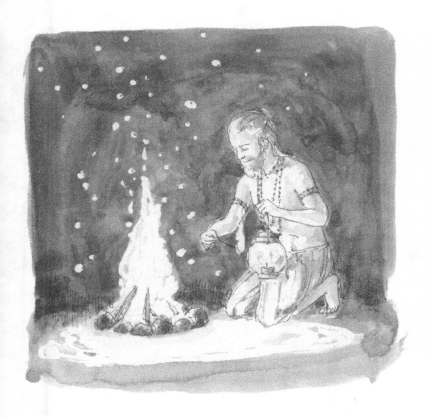

Fig. 16:
According to Yoga, every miniscule vibration in the universe is veiled in varying
proportions by three qualities – *sattva*, *rajas* and *tamas*

The interplay of the veils *sattva*, *rajas* and *tamas* may be thought of as the qualities that metamorphose pure vibrations into the entities of emergent reality. These include our body. Here the veils do not in any way invalidate the fact that the smallest unit of life in our body is the cell and that those cells arise from interacting molecules, which are themselves facilitators of our stories. The veils simply refer to an imaginary hierarchy that churns vibrations within the molecules that facilitate the manifestation of our stories. Accordingly, when that hierarchy consists of an abundance of *tamas*, we embody the darkness of sleepy lethargy; when of *rajas*, the fire of restless activity; and, when of *sattva*, the light of illuminating clarity.

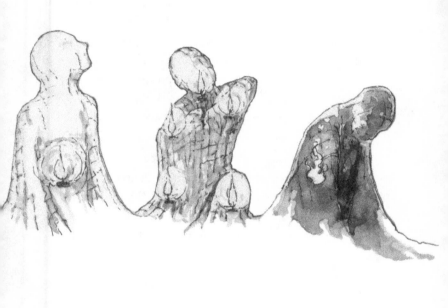

Fig. 17:
The interplay of the three qualities may be seen as that which metamorphoses vibrations
into entities of emergent reality

Having somewhat comprehended the interplay of the veils of *sattva*, *rajas* and *tamas* in relation to our body, we remind ourselves why we did so: to equip ourselves with a way to master the tiny instrument that we are. This mastery provides the self-composure needed to re-chart our trajectory in tandem with the betterment of society. For clarity's sake, let us ground ourselves in the following before we proceed: our body may be seen as the product of an interplay amongst *sattva*, *rajas* and *tamas* that continues and changes in accord with our needs. *Sattva* clarifies those needs. The greater the proportion of *sattva*, the more deftly the veils of *sattva*, *rajas* and *tamas* interplay to satisfy our clarified needs. Let us now proceed to self-mastery.

7
Self-mastery

Our self-mastery is the fine tuning of the tiny instrument that we are. To start, we plant a little *sattva* in ourselves by pondering two entwined strands of knowledge: first, our stories, both inherited and experienced, lie at the heart of the arising of our cells, which then spawn the strings[1] that collectively make our body; second, the consistency and arrangement of those strings determine our body's form. With the aforementioned in mind, we may deduce that our form will reflect our stories. Thus because our stories are unique to us, our form will also be unique to us, invariably meaning that there is no single correct form for our body. There is, however, an optimal equilibrium for its unique form.

[1] For the purpose of this book, string is defined as a unique collection of interrelating cells that form the underlying substance of every tissue, organ and system that collectively comprise our body.

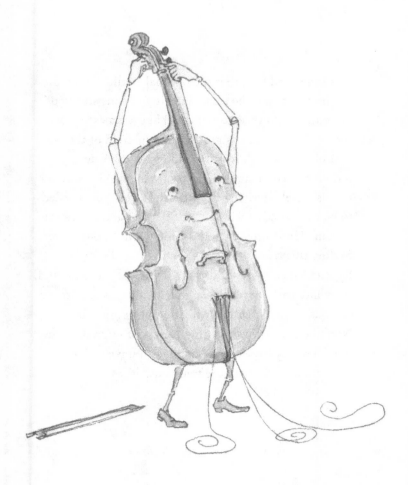

Fig. 18:
Our self-mastery is the fine tuning of the tiny instrument that we are

It is suggested here that the optimal equilibrium for our body is when the arrangement and consistency of our strings allows us to stand tall like a majestic tree, rooted deep in Earth's ground and unafraid of the wind that blows through its surrounding space. A deeply rooted tree commands the capacity to stabilise and nourish itself, deriving from Earth the support needed to be composed as it weathers the wind and reaches to the sun. Unfortunately, amidst the winds of our lives, finding this tree in us can be a challenge. Before we have a chance to establish support from Earth's ground, the wind, with its ever-changing conditions and its devious unpredictability, will attempt to unsettle us. Nonetheless, however stormy, listless or unpredictable the wind may be, we must strive with unwavering conviction to discover the tree in us.

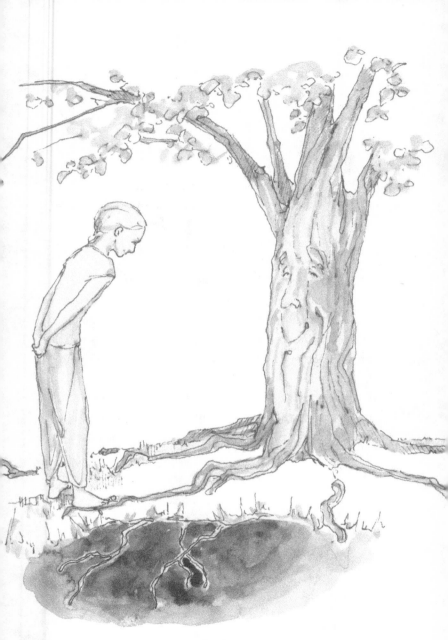

Fig. 19:
A tree that is deeply rooted in Earth's ground commands the capacity
to stabilise and nourish itself

We may find this inner tree by invigorating our cells through learning simple life practices: for example, how to eat mindfully, move gracefully and stand surely[2]. By eating mindfully, we nourish the vitality of our strings. By moving gracefully, we encourage the malleability of our strings. And by standing surely, we fortify the durability of our strings. If we go about these lessons uninterruptedly and with devotion over a prolonged period of time, the fruits of our efforts support us to breathe peacefully through our actions and to sit quietly in our contemplations. This, in turn, develops the *sattva* we had previously planted, creating a light that permeates our every cell, illuminating to us our stories embedded deep within them. We become acquainted with our inner self.

[2] For suggestions that may support each of the practices, please refer to Appendices I, II and III, respectively.

In being acquainted with our inner self, we are also granted knowledge of our fortitudes and fragilities. This is central to our self-mastery because it equips us with the means to withstand the wind as we strive to become the tree within us. For example, if the wind is stormy, we use our fortitudes to collect ourselves so our fragilities do not succumb to the wind that is whirling us around. Similarly, if the wind is lethargic, we also use our fortitudes, but this time to reignite the embers of hope and purpose that are still faintly glowing within our fragilities, invigorating ourselves so the wind has no chance to wear us down toward the ground. In short, we draw on our inner self to transcend the flux of the wind by mastering our response to it.

The capacity to transcend the wind has a profound effect on our brain. It serves to calm the turbulent flow of the brain's rivers, giving them a chance to form new associations among themselves and to discover caverns of treasure deep within its hills and valleys. This – the reader may recall from Chapter 3 – encourages change in the fine structures of our brain, a change that results in a new narrative being served up. Because this new narrative results from our striving for our inner tree, the narrative steers us into a self-conduct that reflects the composure of a tree, which, in turn, causes our cells to increasingly spawn strings with an arrangement and material consistency supportive of such conduct. We start to embody a tree that is calibrated with Earth's ground and at ease with the fluxes of the surrounding space.

8
Creativity

We approached the subject of self-mastery by drawing inspiration from the composure of a tree. However, on closer scrutiny of the tree, it is apparent that in addition to its healthy relationship with both Earth's ground and the surrounding space, it also joyously and unassumingly blossoms into the surrounding space. A tree is not only unafraid of the wind: it also harnesses the wind to make music with its leaves, expressing life. By virtue of its expressive blossoming, a tree's sprawling branches provide shelter for nesters and lovers alike. Whether it's the chirping birds nesting on its branches or the crooning lovers below, a tree, by expressing its life, also encourages the rest of life to thrive. Considering this beautiful miracle, it naturally follows that we now turn to our own expressivity.

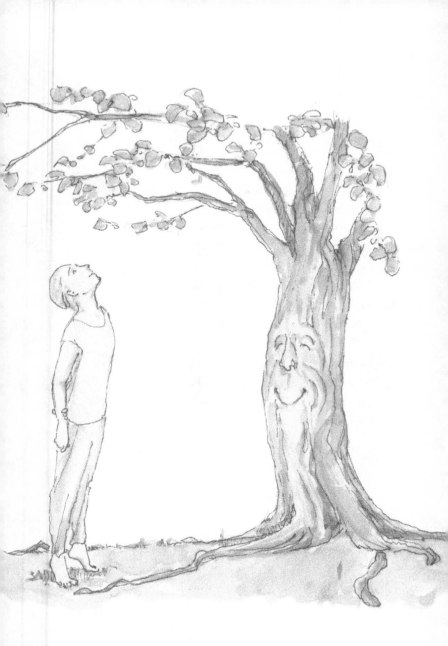

Fig. 20:
A tree, in addition to being at ease with the surrounding space, also joyously and
unassumingly blossoms into it

If we quiet ourselves, we may sense how our heart rhythmically beats and how our blood gently leaps, both of which are a result of our interacting cells. We may also sense how the expansion and contraction of our breath is a dance of our various strings working in concert. These varied sensations are testimonies to the fact that the life within us is in continuous movement. When these movements become imbued with the narrative of our brain, they transform into an expression. Because we are unequivocally dependent on our brain to comport ourselves through life, it is suggested here that we are innately expressive. We are expressive social beings.

As expressive social beings, it would be prudent to know that expressions are principally actions. This means that our every expression is bound to the laws of cause and effect. In obedience to these laws, our expressions will have repercussions. With this in mind, as a tiny instrument whose spirit is to encourage harmony in our interactions, we ought to refrain from compulsive expressions. Such expressions have the potential to result in untoward repercussions, constraining the potential for harmony in our interactions. In the hope of minimising this wasteful constraint, it is suggested here that we channel our innate need for expression into works of creation.

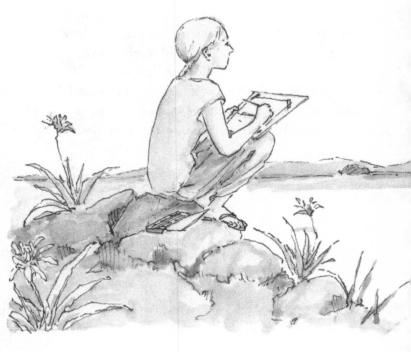

Fig. 21:
A work of creation may be seen as a statement of who we are
at a specific point in time

A work of creation may be seen as a statement of who we are at a specific point in time. It may take the form of colour on paper or arrangements of melodic notes, but it is by no means limited to these. It can be any idea that, in our efforts to formulate and manifest it, claims our all; the only caveat being that in our doing so, we knowingly cause no one to fall. It should also exude originality. For this, we may simply draw on the fact that we each have a unique story, infusing into our creations the lights of joy and shadows of sorrow associated with our story. Should our creation enchant humanity into a reflective reverie, we would have made our story a gift to society.

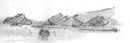

Irrespective of our story enchanting society, the freedom we may feel through the act of creating satisfies our innate need for expression, granting us an internal contentment that steers us away from the haste of compulsive expressions, reducing the probability of untoward repercussions. It also balances the introspective discipline associated with our earlier self-mastery. The reconciliation of these two somewhat contrasting but mutually complementary forces – creativity and self-mastery – supports our body to settle into an equilibrium that is now not only calibrated with Earth's ground and the surrounding space, but also centred in relation to objects that pervade the surrounding space. We start to be in that state which a tree sacredly embodies – equanimity.

9
Unity

The previous two chapters – Self-mastery and Creativity – suggested how, by yoking our inherited story and our experienced stories, we may cultivate ourselves to be in equanimity. For clarity's sake, let us recapitulate the essence of both chapters and their synergy: through the sweat and tears of self-mastery, we support every string of our body to be in tune with every other. Through the liberty that comes with creativity, we cajole those harmoniously tuned strings to feel unrestrained yet measured in their expression. Together, self-mastery and creativity, if embraced uninterruptedly and wholeheartedly, tunes the strings of the tiny instrument that we are so that it – and we – are in a state of equanimity.

In a state of equanimity, we are granted the strength of self-composure that benefits us with the capacity to be sensitive to the consequences of our actions. This sensitivity enables us to somewhat anticipate the multiple effects of our every action, positioning us to positively influence the far-reaching and ever-intricate workings of cause and effect that characterise emergent reality. Should we choose to apply our capacity for sensitivity to our interactions, we would, in effect, be harmonising ourselves with other entities of emergent reality. It is suggested here that this harmony, together with an overarching concern for the welfare of society, re-charts our collective trajectory.

Closer to ourselves, a sensitivity to the consequences of our actions supports attention to new sensations. These include sensations associated with events both within and around the spatial boundary of our body. Sensing these events, we may appreciate how events around us are entwined with events within us, all obeying the laws of cause and effect, just as actions do. Appreciating events in this way, we may grasp the futility of plotting and controlling events around us. Instead, we are awakened to the joy of observing how events within us – the quivers of our gut, the beats of our heart and the evenness of our breath – respond to events around us, using these observations to guide the instrumentation of our budding actions. It is suggested here that it is in observing before acting that we re-chart our individual trajectory.

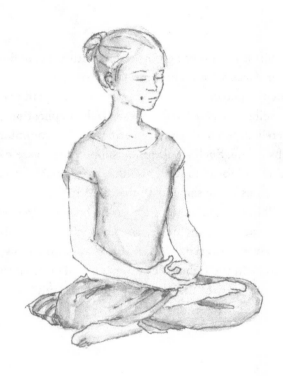

Fig. 22:
Attention to new sensations allows us to observe how events within us
respond to events around us

By virtue of observing how events within us are finely interwoven with events around us, we may progressively come to perceive that the diversity of emergent reality, as well as its associated disorder and complications, are merely different degrees of perfection of a common substratum. Such a perception supports us to see past name and form, to recognise that that which is deep within us is the same in all that is. Whether in the spellbinding grandeur of a clear night sky or the gentle cow that roams the fields, we may begin to recognise ourselves in everything else. This recognition allows us to be in the richness of diversity, while feeling the tranquil unity of that diversity. Put succinctly, we are liberated to live as one.

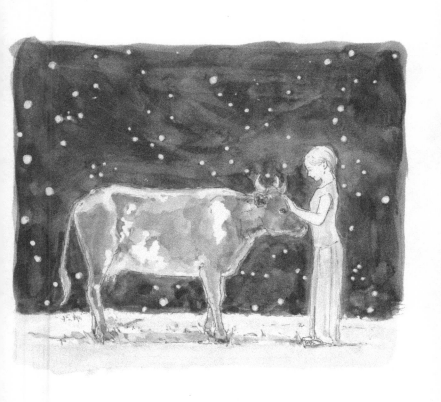

Fig. 23:
In seeing beyond name and form, we may perhaps recognise
ourselves in everything else

Should we feel our uniting oneness, a number of questions may arise. At the end of our life, would the phenomenon that gives life to the substratum within the spatial boundary of our body cease to exist or is it a moving soul that keeps a record of our body's actions and reactions, using that record to guide itself towards a suitable new body? If the latter, how does this moving soul liberate itself from the cycle of birth and death? And, if it should find liberation, does this soul retain its individuality or does it merge with the soul of all? The unravelling of these mindboggling questions is another story. But whatever the answers, we are today a tiny instrument in an unfathomably grand orchestra. While the primordial origins of this orchestra remain a mystery, its symphony depends upon our feeling its unity.

Appendix I

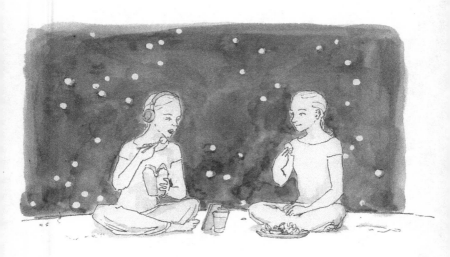

Ayurveda

as a means to eating mindfully

Eating is the taking in of food that provides nutrients that are used by our body. Our bodies being unique, food suitable for one body may not necessarily be suitable for another. We ought to be mindful of this point and make every effort to ingest food compatible with the uniqueness of our body. We should also ensure that our eating of that food pleasures and soothes both the senses of our body and the rivers of our brain. Such a relationship with food can be found embedded in the wisdom of a tradition originating out of Ancient India – Ayurveda.

At the very heart of Ayurveda is the notion that our body – and environment – are governed by three principles of unique qualities. They are: *vata*, *pitta* and *kapha*. These principles may be thought of as permutations of the veiled vibrations that we fundamentally are. The relative proportions of the three are determined at the moment of our conception. As we grow, develop and age, those proportions adapt to the corresponding needs of our body and brain in relation to our environment. This includes the nine months we were in our mother's womb.

When the proportions of *vata*, *pitta* and *kapha* within us adapt in harmony with that of our environment, we are said to be in a state of balance. Such a state, however, is continuously challenged. The forces of our environment can aggravate the forces within us, churning our intrinsic proportions of *vata*, *pitta* and *kapha* away from that which supports balance – we can become imbalanced, and consequently, prone to illness. To manage our propensity for imbalance, Ayurveda recommends consulting a practitioner trained in its wisdom.

A consultation with an Ayurvedic practitioner entails the taking of our life history, an appreciation of our current diet and lifestyle, the taking of our pulse, a visual analysis of our tongue and face, and at times, an inspection of our faeces. This is how the practitioner deciphers our uniqueness in terms of *vata*, *pitta* and *kapha*. Drawing on that insight, the practitioner formulates a programme that, if embraced, encourages the proportions of *vata*, *pitta* and *kapha* within us into proportions that support our being in a state of balance.

The programme is multilayered in nature and almost always includes guidance relating to eating: how to choose foods compatible with the uniqueness of our body, how to choose food suitable for our age and life circumstance, how to adapt our choice of food to seasonal variations, the manner in which food should be prepared, as well as how and when that food should be ingested. Should we take heed of that guidance, applying it to our eating, we would in effect live our way into the practice of eating mindfully.

Appendix II

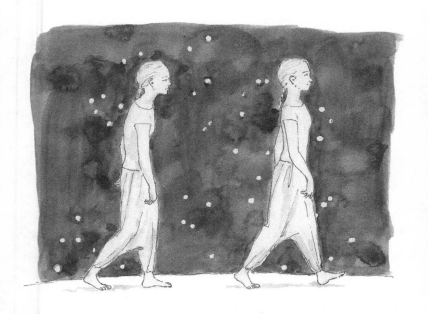

Movement Integration

as a means to moving gracefully

We volitionally move by recruiting our body's muscles to change their location in space. That recruitment is coordinated by our brain. More often than not, our brain incites the same combination of muscles to be enlisted. This creates patterns in our movement. While the patterns are undoubtedly a necessity, should they cause our movement to feel forced or rigid, or cause us to feel inhibited, it would serve us to modulate those patterns to our betterment.

Before we attempt to modulate our movement patterns, it would help to know that although our brain coordinates the recruitment of our muscles, that coordination is regulated. It is regulated by our body's sense of orientation to the Earth's ground and our body's sense of orientation to the surrounding space. These somewhat opposing senses give rise to bodily sensations which are used by our muscles to self-organise around. This means our patterns of movement are a function of both our brain and the self-organisation of our muscles.

The key to modulating our movement patterns is attention to the sensations associated with the self-organisation of our muscles. In practice, this starts with tuning in to the sensations as they arise. This can be challenging, however, as the sensations tend to be masked by habits that characterise the very patterns we wish to modulate. In other words, our habits deprive us of feeling the wholeness of arising sensations. To transcend this challenge, we need to be aware of our habits, and to do so, we may benefit from a method.

One method that resonates with the spirit of this book can be found in the works of Caryn McHose and Kevin Frank, beautifully presented through their book: *How Life Moves*. Their method consists of a series of explorative exercises that use an abbreviation of our evolutionary story as a metaphor. The exercises serve to internalise in the person doing them a foundational notion of their method: preparation for movement. According to McHose and Frank, embedded in our preparation for movement are our habits.

As per the aforementioned method, by repeatedly observing our preparation for movement, we may become progressively aware of our habits. This awareness allows us to feel through our habits as we move, positioning us to tune in to the arising of sensations associated with the self-organisation of our muscles. Should we, in tuning in, also be spatially curious while ensuring we remain connected with ground, doing so in a state of composed slowness, we would in effect be cajoling our brain into integrating those sensations with itself. This lies at the heart of modulating our movement patterns – a modulation that paves the way to our moving gracefully.

Appendix III

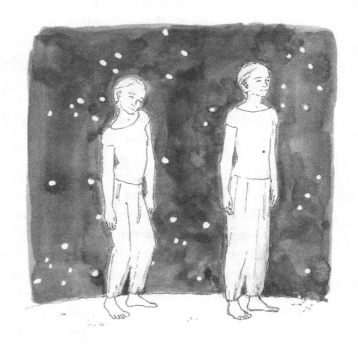

Structural Integration

as a means to standing surely

We stand by recruiting our body's muscles to transcend Earth's gravitational pull on us. This recruitment is coordinated by our brain. More often than not, our brain incites the same combination of muscles to be enlisted. This creates tensional patterns in our standing. Without these patterns we would collapse. Even so, should we be feeling unsteady in our standing, then there is a chance that our tensional patterns have caused our body to be in tensional disequilibrium.

Tensional disequilibrium manifests through a tissue called fascia. This tissue is found around and within our muscles and is continuous with the membranes that envelop our visceral chambers. Fascia, broadly speaking, is composed of two types of fibres of varying proportions: collagen and elastin. The ratio of collagen to elastin depends on the functional demand on an area of our body. A part of our body that stabilises us would have a greater proportion of collagen than a part of our body that frequently changes its shape.

When our body is in tensional disequilibrium, the proportions of collagen and elastin fibres in various parts of our body deviate from that which is healthy. This deviation gives rise to compensatory tension in other parts and layers of our body, which, in turn, may cause our muscles to be unnecessarily tense or create constrictions within our visceral chambers. Our body becomes somewhat disorganised, challenging our ability to stand with ease. To overcome this challenge, it would help to reorganise our body.

Should we choose to reorganise our body, we may benefit from a little helper. One such helper is someone who practices Structural Integration, a method pioneered by a remarkable woman who was ahead of her time: Dr Ida Rolf. A practitioner of her method understands the ins and outs of fascia, and draws on this knowledge to reorganise our body. He or she employs that understanding in such a way that our body is guided to derive stability from Earth's ground in order to healthily relate to the surrounding space.

In practice, a practitioner of Structural Integration begins by taking stock of our tensional patterns. Informed by that knowledge, he or she reorganises our body by applying gentle but deep and sustained pressure on our skin, feeling through our many layers of tissue to arrive at our fascia. Once in touch with our fascia, the practitioner cajoles its underlying fibres of collagen and elastin to return to a healthy ratio. This cascades a chain of events that, in slowly unfolding, nurtures our body into a tensional equilibrium that is supportive of our standing surely.

Afterword

I came into this world through parents of Sri Lankan descent, taking my first breath on a winter morning in Aberdeen, Scotland. Roughly two years later, I found myself in multicultural Malaysia. It was in the tropics of Malaysia that I was raised and where my development was nourished by my unrestrained indulgence of bowel-moving papayas and cell-hydrating coconuts.

A defining factor of my development were weekends at the home of my grandma and grandpa. I would wake up to the sound of grandma doing her prayers where, in trance-like fashion, she would sing with utter devotion to depictions of Hindu gods carefully placed upon her altar. I would respectfully, but agitatedly, observe her, as I was impatient for what came after.

When grandma finished her prayers, we would adjourn to the kitchen. There, using batter lovingly prepared by grandpa to the finest consistency, she would make my favourite breakfast – a savoury pancake-like crepe called "dosa". My mouth watering, I would gleefully gobble one dosa after another, savouring its fine flavours in my mouth. And as I freely stuffed my mouth, grandma would enthral me with stories whose characters were the very same gods she had sung to a few hours earlier.

The stories were often themed along the lines of good prevailing over evil through the application of deep wisdom. Hanging on to every word grandma

spoke, those stories made indelible impressions on
me. So much so that to this very day, I try to emulate
the good in the stories. I do not always succeed, but
I try. As impactful as those stories were on me, and
as thoroughly as I enjoyed them, I had one gnawing
concern. Who created those gods that grandma spoke
about so vividly and assuredly? As grandma didn't have
an adequate answer, I posed that question to the gods
on her altar. Despite my repeated attempts, and despite
the best behaviour my mischievous young self could
muster, they never answered.

Not knowing where the gods came from frustrated me
as a child. I found it absurd that adults around me made
such a hullaballoo – rituals in temples, observances of
auspicious days, etc. – around gods whose origins they
could not convincingly explain. Fortunately for my
sanity, I made peace with not knowing. After all, there
was no real need to know, for I was feeling happily alive
and I was being showered with unconditional love.
Not just from grandma and grandpa, but also from
my aunts, uncles, cousins and, of course, my treasured
nuclear family. I am forever thankful for all the love
that was bestowed upon me so warmly and freely as a
child.

*

As I left the innocence of childhood and ventured
into the muddle of adulthood, my development took

a progression that was somewhat typical of the strata of society I found myself in: I finished high school, went to university and began salaried employment afterwards. The course of landing that employment, however, requires some expansion, for embedded in it are seeds that would germinate and blossom as I matured.

To land a salaried job, one typically has to write an application. In my case, I wrote countless applications. Despite the sheer numbers, every one of them was rejected. Disheartened and in dire straits to earn a living, I resorted to waiting tables and washing dishes. The emotions associated with this unforeseen necessity, compounded by matters of the heart running amuck at that time, caused me to feel rather low. Downtrodden by forces outside my sphere of direct control, I gravitated towards the soothing yet powerful verses of the Bhagavad-Gita, a philosophical text of Indic origin. The version I read was without commentary.

I knew of the Bhagavad-Gita as a child because it stood prominently in our family home. But it was only in my dejection that I delved into its wisdom. As I meditated on its verses and contemplated their meaning, a fire was ignited in me. That fire illuminated to me the trivialness of my melancholy and galvanised me to become a warrior who commanded the composure of an astute diplomat. Energised and clear-headed, I began to find joy in washing dishes till they were squeaky clean and in disarming the odd pompous customer with my firm smile. Curiously enough, just as I was embracing life in this way, I received a letter offering me a post at an international consultancy based in the city of London. I took it.

*

When I began employment in London, I was enthusiastic and ever raring to go. After all, the journey there had been far from smooth and I was feeling very thankful. But then something unexpected happened. Despite succeeding in the challenges that came with the job, and despite its many perks, my enthusiasm quickly waned. I found myself craving purpose and meaning, neither of which were to be found in my job at the consultancy. So after much brooding, I decided to do something about it. I walked gingerly to my boss's office and asked him if I could take a mini-sabbatical: I wanted to volunteer with an organisation based in Rwanda. To my surprise, he granted my wish. A few months later, I was on a plane to Kigali, the capital of Rwanda.

Among the things I did in Rwanda was help a group of women brainstorm projects that would improve their livelihoods. We discussed the details whilst sitting on the green grass of their village, which was located on the outskirts of Kigali. Most of the women I was with had witnessed the horrors of the Rwandan genocide first-hand and had one painful thing in common: they were all HIV+ and, more often than not, had contracted it through domestic violence. Their capacity for resilience, despite the weight they were unfairly made to carry, moved me in a very profound way.

In meeting with these women, I found myself thinking about their situation. Through my reflections and observations, I came to the following understanding: the women's situation derived from a social fabric that had been gruesomely tattered by the genocide. The genocide, in turn, had been orchestrated by men who infused fear into the divisive structures of Rwandan society, which itself was a legacy of a former colonial power with a greedy agenda. Thus, I concluded that the injustice of their situation had roots in greed and fear.

After my mini-sabbatical was over and I was back in London, the far-reaching consequences of actions stemming from greed and fear consumed my thoughts and led to me making a pact with myself: I would always strive to keep the permutations of greed and fear at bay and, where possible, work towards the obliteration of its evil manifestations. After much reading, I decided I could realise my pact best by enlisting myself in the fight against poverty and inequality. So after roughly five years at the London firm, I resigned.

*

I tend to be thorough in anything I do. The fight against poverty and inequality was no different. Fully aware that I had much to learn before going into battle, I decided to get a feel for the fight by embarking on a fellowship with a San Francisco-based organisation called Kiva. The fellowship assigned me to Zimbabwe, where – squashed into dilapidated busses and huddled in the back of pickup trucks – I travelled throughout the beautiful countryside. My task was to further Kiva's mission of expanding financial access to underserved communities throughout Zimbabwe. I succeeded at my task, but only because my hand was gently held by the ever-charismatic Zimbabweans I worked with. I had the time of my life and the memories are dear to my heart.

On completion of my fellowship with Kiva, I moved to Edinburgh. Nourished by the beauty of that city, and feeling incubated by the intellectual richness of its main university, I earned a master's degree in Sustainable Energy, writing my dissertation on rural development through improved energy services. After completion of this degree, I was truly ready to join the good fight. As the fight consisted of many varied and fundamentally different battles, I chose a battle on the island of Borneo. The battle had long been raging and was spearheaded by a local grassroots organisation called Tonibung.

Tonibung's mission was to train marginalised indigenous communities to build and maintain renewable energy schemes to power their remote villages, which were often located deep in the forest. The electrification of their villages would allow them to have access to an amenity many of us take for granted – light for reading. I supported Tonibung's mission by applying insights derived from my master's degree to their efforts. As we worked together, I became increasingly awed by the skill and innovativeness of the warriors in Borneo. Just like the Zimbabweans, they had highly effective solutions to their unique problems. They barely needed my input.

Awed by the raw talent at Tonibung, it dawned on me that Tonibung, as well as many other grassroots initiatives around the world, could do without the haughty patronisation that often characterises foreign involvement. Organisations such as Tonibung may certainly benefit from new technological know-how and associated training, but assuming they have access to equitable financial capital, they are usually self-sufficient. What they did need, however, was for society to stop encroaching on their lives. In the case of Borneo, they needed the construction of huge dams to be halted and for deforestation to be prevented, both of which can be achieved through the choices each and every one of us makes.

Along with the realisation that my role in the battle at Borneo was not as significant as my ego would have liked, I recognised that I lacked one crucial ingredient: passion for that particular battle. While my work ethic was hard to fault, and while I certainly had the mental strength to stay the course, I didn't have zeal. Unlike my friends at Tonibung, who were fervently fighting for their people and their right to survive, my role was merely a job. All well and good if that satisfied me. But I wanted more. I wanted to feel passion in what I did. So, accepting this hard truth, I bowed out of the battle at Borneo.

*

On bowing out, it occurred to me that I had enlisted as a soldier in the fight against poverty and inequality not because I had a visceral calling, but because I was unfulfilled with consulting in London. In other words, my motivation for joining the fight was fundamentally flawed. This was not to say I have any regrets, for that could not be further away from the truth. I did, however, need to rethink my part in the fight – and whatever that part would be, in addition to battling the vicissitudes of greed and fear, it had to incite passion in me. With this in mind, and to guide myself towards such a part, I took stock of myself.

In taking stock of myself, I was happy to find that I am a person who feels love at the core of his being and has a strong sense of right and wrong. I use that sense to guide my actions. I am aware that my right may be another's wrong and vice versa, so when I act, I draw on the love that I feel in my core and infuse it into my actions. I hope my actions bring a quality that furthers what is right for the collective good.

Love in the name of good is easier said than done – because as pure as love may be, as it moves through one's body and into one's actions, it gets somewhat corrupted by the story embedded in the body. This is certainly the case with me. My stocktaking revealed that my story included a number of idiosyncrasies, some of which are harmless and some of which have a degree of ruthlessness. This discovery made me realise that the love I infuse into my actions may not be as pure as I imagine it to be. Pondering this revelation, I figured I would be able to minimise the corruption of love flowing through me if ensured I always felt free.

Freedom is multi-layered and – as William Cowper says – has a thousand charms to show. Be that as it may, as human beings who need sustenance, freedom's charms tend to hinge on one's basic needs being met first. I had no wish to live in a remote cave, surviving through hunting and gathering, and I did not want to return to the mundaneness of salaried employment or venture into the tedium of grant writing – both of which would result in my unfreedom – so I honed in on a new means to satisfy my basic needs, one in which the world would also be my oyster. I became a practitioner of Structural Integration, a form of manual therapy.

*

I felt purpose and meaning in this practice. Delighted to feel sentiments that I had long been yearning for, I was eager to evolve my practice of Structural Integration into a craft. This demanded that I not only refine my technical skills, but also be centred in myself. Only in being centred would I have the perceptual clarity to sensitively tune in to the subtleties of the person I was working with and negotiate traces of greed and fear that may have scarred them unknowingly. Furthermore, it was my duty: if a person was going to trust me with handling their body, I had to be in tune with mine first.

With the benefit of hindsight, I can see that this self-centring had begun when I first read the Bhagavad-Gita. But as wise and soothing at its verses were, it had not expanded on the practicalities of being centred. It was towards these practicalities that I now focussed my efforts. I embodied the philosophy underpinning Structural Integration and started to embrace a number of daily practices. Among others, these included mindfulness in my eating and a modulation of my movement patterns, both of which are deepened through my commitment to a consistent Hatha Yoga practice.

Through my devotion to practices that nurtured my centring, the composite of animated matter who I was settled in an equilibrium of tranquil calm. Relishing the sweetness of this state, something unexpected happened: passion emerged in my body. I harnessed it and became progressively more aware of the forces behind my very existence. Reflecting on this awareness, I decided to describe them by writing this book.

The process of writing of this book has been sheer joy and has allowed me to feel like a covert agent in the fight for a more equitable society. I am indebted to the many opportunities that facilitated this privileged feeling.

Raveen Kulenthran
Munich, January 2022

Bibliography

I have organised this bibliography according to each chapter in this book, and the books that inspired and fed into each chapter. However, due to the holistic nature of the subject matter, the impact of each listed book extends into each and every chapter. I am eternally indebted to the authors listed below.

1: A Wrinkled Crinkle
The Big Picture: On the Origins of Life, Meaning and the Universe Itself
by Sean Carrol
Dutton, New York, 2017

The Fabric of the Cosmos: Space, Time, and the Texture of Reality
by Brian Greene
Vintage Books, New York, 2004

A Brief History of Time
by Stephen Hawking
Bantam Press, London, 1988

War and Peace
by Leo Tolstoy
Oxford University Press, New York, 2010

2: Inherited Story
What is Life?
by Erwin Schrödinger
Cambridge University Press, Cambridge, 2018

The Mysterious World of the Human Genome: How Genetics and Epigenetics Make Us What We Are
by Frank Ryan
William Collins, London, 2016

The Developing Genome: An Introduction to Behavioral Epigenetics
by David S. Moore
Oxford University Press, New York, 2017

Why Evolution is True
by Jerry A. Coyne
Oxford University Press, New York, 2010

How Life Moves: Exploration in Meaning and Body Awareness
by Caryn McHose and Kevin Frank
North Atlantic Books, Berkeley, 2006

3: Experienced Stories
The Brain: The Story of You
by David Eagleman
Canongate Books, Edinburgh, 2016

The Brain that Changes Itself: Stories of Personal Triumph from the Frontiers of Brain Science
by Norman Doidge
Penguin Books, London, 2008

The Brain's Way of Healing: Stories of Remarkable Recoveries and Discoveries
by Norman Doidge
Penguin Books, London, 2016

Medical Neurobiology
by Peggy Mason
Oxford University Press, New York, 2011

The Science of Fate: Why Your Future is More Predictable Than You Think
by Hannah Critchlow
Hodder & Stoughton, London, 2019

4: Society
Identity and Violence: The Illusion of Destiny
by Amartya Sen
Penguin Books, London, 2017

Development as Freedom
by Amartya Sen
Oxford University Press, New York, 2001

Media Control: The Spectacular Achievements of Propaganda
by Noam Chomsky
Seven Stories Press, New York, 2002

The Prize: The Epic Quest for Oil, Money and Power
by Daniel Yiergin
Simon & Schuster, New York, 2009

*King Leopold's Ghost: A Story of Greed, Terror and Heroism in Colonial Afric*a
by Adam Hochschild
Pan Macmillan, Basingstoke, 2006

5: A Tiny Instrument
Emotional Anatomy
by Stanley Keleman
Center Press, Berkeley, 1985

Job's Body: A Handbook for Bodywork
by Deane Juhan
Station Hill Press, Barrytown, 2003

The Woodlanders
by Thomas Hardy
Oxford University Press, New York, 2009

6: A Leaf Out of India
*The Argumentative Indian: Writings on Indian Culture,
History and Identity*
by Amartya Sen
Penguin Books, London, 2006

The Bhagavad Gita: Translated with an Introduction
by Juan Mascaró
Penguin Books India, Haryana, 2009

7: Self-mastery
*The Mirror of Yoga: Awakening the Intelligence of
Body and Mind*
by Richard Freeman
Shambhala Publications, Boulder, 2010

*The Yoga Sūtras of Patañjali: A New Edition,
Translation, and Commentary*
by Edwin F. Bryant
North Point Press, New York, 2009

Ayurvedic Healing: A Comprehensive Guide
by David Frawley
Lotus Press, 2001

*Functional Anatomy of Yoga: A Guide for Practitioners
and Teachers*
by David Keil
Lotus Publishing, Chichester, 2014

Fascial and Membrane Technique
by Peter Schwind
Elsevier, London, 2006

*Fascial Fitness: How to be Resilient, Elegant and
Dynamic in Everyday Life and Sport*
by Robert Schleip
Lotus Publishing, Chichester, 2014

8: Creativity
Sadhana: The Realisation of Life
by Rabindranath Tagore
Tradition GmbH, Hamburg, 2019

Letters to a Young Poet
by Rainer Maria Rilke
Vintage Books, New York, 1984

9: Unity
*The Upanishads: Translations from the Sanskrit with an
Introduction*
by Juan Mascaró
Penguin Books, London, 2005

Acknowledgements

I am grateful to every person who, through honest discussion, shaped the thoughts that made this book. Persons who come to mind include Romila Kulenthran, Liew Yew Wen, Chan Wei Jun, Gerald Tee, Kenneth Yong, Nicholas Soo, Kantha Ruban, Sutheshan Shanmugarajah, Hesbon Njane Njuguna, Azi Mohamed, Paul Cooke, Adam Petritsis, Sudarshan Ratnavelu, Eftihia Yiannakis, Sebastian Le Scraigne, Wenu Perera, Richard Price, Frank Chouraqui, Anna Pelekanou, Matthew Wellard, Naomi Jones, Aleksandra Paterek, Horacio Cuenca, Kate Ashcroft, Basar Korkankorkmaz, Zoe Green, Ryan Spielman, Pamhidzai Mhongera, Amy Doffegnies, Ganesh Upadhay, Adrian Lasimbang, Gabriel Sundoro Wynn, Grazyna Topolska, Gergana Lambreva, Brigitte Smith, Richard Smith, Anise Smith, Konrad Obermeier, Michael Schabort, Nadja Labudda, Peter Cudek, Katrin Pichl, Stefanie Reichelt and Berivan Kaya. I apologize to those whose names I have inadvertently left out. I am especially grateful to Liam Robertson, Brigitte Smith, Amy Doffegnies and Anna Barret, who read and critiqued the manuscript. I am indebted to the illustrator, Asta Caplan. Her ability to create with childlike perfection touches me deeply. I am also grateful to my editor, Howard Fine, who has mastered the art of correcting without changing. I am thankful to Nerina Wilter, who so carefully designed this book. Last but not least, I am forever thankful for the unconditional and unwavering love that my parents, Kulenthran Arumugam and Thayanithi Ponnudurai, have bestowed upon me. Their love keeps me whole.

About the Author

Raveen Kulenthran is a practitioner of Structural Integration, a form of manual therapy. He holds a Master of Engineering from the University of Nottingham and a Master of Science from the University of Edinburgh. He spends any free time he has pondering what truth is. He lives in Munich, Germany.

CPSIA information can be obtained
at www.ICGtesting.com
Printed in the USA
BVHW042138310822
646047BV00001B/2

9 783982 427324